THIS PLANNER BELONGS TO

Contact:

BIRTHDAYS & DATES TO REMEMBER

Birthdays

Dates to Remember

DATE	WHO	DATE	EVENT

"Look past your thoughts, so you may drink the pure nectar of This Moment."

—RUMI

MINDFULNESS
priorities

Monday	*Tuesday*	*Wednesday*

LET GO OF YOUR MIND, AND THEN BE MINDFUL. CLOSE YOUR EYES AND LISTEN!

–Rumi

NOTES

Thursday	*Friday*	*Saturday*	*Sunday*

BIRTHDAYS

MINDFULNESS *intentions*

NOTES

	Monday	*Tuesday*	*Wednesday*
ACTIVITIES			
FOCUS			
MINDFULNESS			

TRACKER

	M	T	W	T	F	S	S
	○	○	○	○	○	○	○
	○	○	○	○	○	○	○
	○	○	○	○	○	○	○
	○	○	○	○	○	○	○
	○	○	○	○	○	○	○

Thursday	*Friday*	*Saturday*	*Sunday*

REFLECTIONS

JOY	CHALLENGES	MOOD	LEARNINGS

MINDFULNESS *intentions*

	Monday	*Tuesday*	*Wednesday*
ACTIVITIES			
FOCUS			
MINDFULNESS			

NOTES

TRACKER	M	T	W	T	F	S	S
	○	○	○	○	○	○	○
	○	○	○	○	○	○	○
	○	○	○	○	○	○	○
	○	○	○	○	○	○	○
	○	○	○	○	○	○	○

Thursday	*Friday*	*Saturday*	*Sunday*

REFLECTIONS

JOY	CHALLENGES	MOOD	LEARNINGS

MINDFULNESS
intentions

NOTES

	Monday	*Tuesday*	*Wednesday*
ACTIVITIES			
FOCUS			
MINDFULNESS			

TRACKER	M	T	W	T	F	S	S
	○	○	○	○	○	○	○
	○	○	○	○	○	○	○
	○	○	○	○	○	○	○
	○	○	○	○	○	○	○
	○	○	○	○	○	○	○

Thursday	Friday	Saturday	Sunday

REFLECTIONS

JOY	CHALLENGES	MOOD	LEARNINGS

MINDFULNESS *intentions*

NOTES

	Monday	Tuesday	Wednesday
ACTIVITIES			
FOCUS			
MINDFULNESS			

TRACKER	M	T	W	T	F	S	S

Thursday	*Friday*	*Saturday*	*Sunday*

REFLECTIONS

JOY	CHALLENGES	MOOD	LEARNINGS

MINDFULNESS *intentions*

NOTES

	Monday	Tuesday	Wednesday
ACTIVITIES			
FOCUS			
MINDFULNESS			

TRACKER

	M	T	W	T	F	S	S
	○	○	○	○	○	○	○
	○	○	○	○	○	○	○
	○	○	○	○	○	○	○
	○	○	○	○	○	○	○
	○	○	○	○	○	○	○

Thursday	*Friday*	*Saturday*	*Sunday*

REFLECTIONS

JOY	CHALLENGES	MOOD	LEARNINGS

NOTES

"The true secret of happiness lies in taking a genuine interest in all the details of daily life."

—WILLIAM MORRIS

MINDFULNESS
priorities

PARADISE ON EARTH IS WHERE I AM.
–*Voltaire*

Monday	Tuesday	Wednesday

NOTES

Thursday	Friday	Saturday	Sunday

BIRTHDAYS

MINDFULNESS *intentions*

NOTES

	Monday	*Tuesday*	*Wednesday*
ACTIVITIES			
FOCUS			
MINDFULNESS			

TRACKER	M	T	W	T	F	S	S
	○	○	○	○	○	○	○
	○	○	○	○	○	○	○
	○	○	○	○	○	○	○
	○	○	○	○	○	○	○
	○	○	○	○	○	○	○

Thursday	Friday	Saturday	Sunday

REFLECTIONS

JOY	CHALLENGES	MOOD	LEARNINGS

MINDFULNESS *intentions*

NOTES

	Monday	*Tuesday*	*Wednesday*
ACTIVITIES			
FOCUS			
MINDFULNESS			

TRACKER	M	T	W	T	F	S	S
	○	○	○	○	○	○	○
	○	○	○	○	○	○	○
	○	○	○	○	○	○	○
	○	○	○	○	○	○	○
	○	○	○	○	○	○	○

Thursday	Friday	Saturday	Sunday

REFLECTIONS

JOY	CHALLENGES	MOOD	LEARNINGS

MINDFULNESS *intentions*

NOTES

	Monday	Tuesday	Wednesday
ACTIVITIES			
FOCUS			
MINDFULNESS			

TRACKER	M	T	W	T	F	S	S
	○	○	○	○	○	○	○
	○	○	○	○	○	○	○
	○	○	○	○	○	○	○
	○	○	○	○	○	○	○
	○	○	○	○	○	○	○

Thursday	*Friday*	*Saturday*	*Sunday*

REFLECTIONS

JOY	CHALLENGES	MOOD	LEARNINGS

MINDFULNESS *intentions*

	Monday	Tuesday	Wednesday
ACTIVITIES			
FOCUS			
MINDFULNESS			

NOTES

TRACKER	M	T	W	T	F	S	S
	○	○	○	○	○	○	○
	○	○	○	○	○	○	○
	○	○	○	○	○	○	○
	○	○	○	○	○	○	○
	○	○	○	○	○	○	○

Thursday	*Friday*	*Saturday*	*Sunday*

REFLECTIONS

JOY	CHALLENGES	MOOD	LEARNINGS

MINDFULNESS
intentions

NOTES

	Monday	Tuesday	Wednesday
ACTIVITIES			
FOCUS			
MINDFULNESS			

TRACKER	M	T	W	T	F	S	S
	○	○	○	○	○	○	○
	○	○	○	○	○	○	○
	○	○	○	○	○	○	○
	○	○	○	○	○	○	○
	○	○	○	○	○	○	○

Thursday	*Friday*	*Saturday*	*Sunday*

REFLECTIONS

JOY	CHALLENGES	MOOD	LEARNINGS

NOTES

*"In this moment,
there is plenty of time.
In this moment, you are
precisely as you should be.
In this moment there is
infinite possibility."*

— VICTORIA MORAN

MINDFULNESS
priorities

Monday	Tuesday	Wednesday

I DWELL IN POSSIBILITY.
–Emily Dickinson

NOTES

Thursday	Friday	Saturday	Sunday

BIRTHDAYS

MINDFULNESS *intentions*

NOTES

	Monday	Tuesday	Wednesday
ACTIVITIES			
FOCUS			
MINDFULNESS			

TRACKER	M	T	W	T	F	S	S
	○	○	○	○	○	○	○
	○	○	○	○	○	○	○
	○	○	○	○	○	○	○
	○	○	○	○	○	○	○
	○	○	○	○	○	○	○

Thursday	*Friday*	*Saturday*	*Sunday*

REFLECTIONS

JOY	CHALLENGES	MOOD	LEARNINGS

MINDFULNESS *intentions*

	Monday	Tuesday	Wednesday
ACTIVITIES			
FOCUS			
MINDFULNESS			

NOTES

TRACKER	M	T	W	T	F	S	S
	○	○	○	○	○	○	○
	○	○	○	○	○	○	○
	○	○	○	○	○	○	○
	○	○	○	○	○	○	○
	○	○	○	○	○	○	○

Thursday	*Friday*	*Saturday*	*Sunday*

REFLECTIONS

JOY	CHALLENGES	MOOD	LEARNINGS

MINDFULNESS *intentions*

	Monday	*Tuesday*	*Wednesday*
ACTIVITIES			
FOCUS			
MINDFULNESS			

NOTES

TRACKER

	M	T	W	T	F	S	S
	○	○	○	○	○	○	○
	○	○	○	○	○	○	○
	○	○	○	○	○	○	○
	○	○	○	○	○	○	○
	○	○	○	○	○	○	○

Thursday	*Friday*	*Saturday*	*Sunday*

REFLECTIONS

JOY	CHALLENGES	MOOD	LEARNINGS

MINDFULNESS *intentions*

NOTES

	Monday	*Tuesday*	*Wednesday*
ACTIVITIES			
FOCUS			
MINDFULNESS			

TRACKER	M	T	W	T	F	S	S
	○	○	○	○	○	○	○
	○	○	○	○	○	○	○
	○	○	○	○	○	○	○
	○	○	○	○	○	○	○
	○	○	○	○	○	○	○

Thursday	*Friday*	*Saturday*	*Sunday*

REFLECTIONS

JOY	CHALLENGES	MOOD	LEARNINGS

MINDFULNESS *intentions*

	Monday	Tuesday	Wednesday
ACTIVITIES			
FOCUS			
MINDFULNESS			

NOTES

TRACKER	M	T	W	T	F	S	S
	○	○	○	○	○	○	○
	○	○	○	○	○	○	○
	○	○	○	○	○	○	○
	○	○	○	○	○	○	○
	○	○	○	○	○	○	○

Thursday	Friday	Saturday	Sunday

REFLECTIONS

JOY	CHALLENGES	MOOD	LEARNINGS

NOTES

"Forget the past, and live the present hour."

— SARAH KNOWLES BOLTON

MINDFULNESS
priorities

Monday	Tuesday	Wednesday

WHEREVER YOU ARE, BE THERE TOTALLY.
–Eckhart Tolle

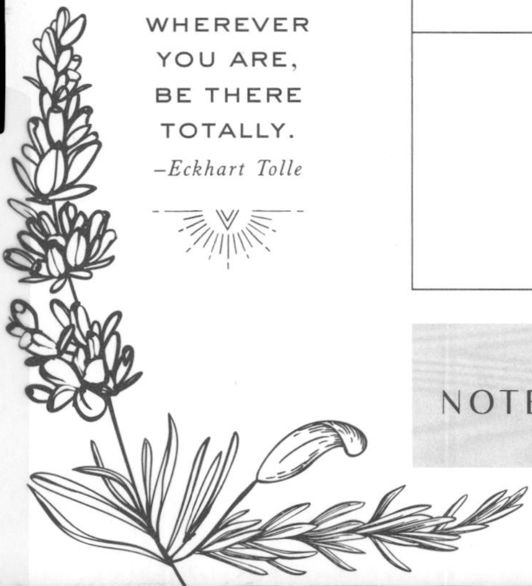

NOTES

Thursday	*Friday*	*Saturday*	*Sunday*

BIRTHDAYS

MINDFULNESS *intentions*

NOTES

	Monday	Tuesday	Wednesday
ACTIVITIES			
FOCUS			
MINDFULNESS			

TRACKER	M	T	W	T	F	S	S

Thursday	Friday	Saturday	Sunday

REFLECTIONS

JOY	CHALLENGES	MOOD	LEARNINGS

MINDFULNESS *intentions*

	Monday	Tuesday	Wednesday
ACTIVITIES			
FOCUS			
MINDFULNESS			

NOTES

TRACKER	M	T	W	T	F	S	S
	○	○	○	○	○	○	○
	○	○	○	○	○	○	○
	○	○	○	○	○	○	○
	○	○	○	○	○	○	○
	○	○	○	○	○	○	○

Thursday	Friday	Saturday	Sunday

REFLECTIONS

JOY	CHALLENGES	MOOD	LEARNINGS

MINDFULNESS
intentions

NOTES

	Monday	Tuesday	Wednesday
ACTIVITIES			
FOCUS			
MINDFULNESS			

TRACKER

	M	T	W	T	F	S	S
	○	○	○	○	○	○	○
	○	○	○	○	○	○	○
	○	○	○	○	○	○	○
	○	○	○	○	○	○	○
	○	○	○	○	○	○	○

Thursday	*Friday*	*Saturday*	*Sunday*

REFLECTIONS

JOY	CHALLENGES	MOOD	LEARNINGS

MINDFULNESS *intentions*

NOTES

	Monday	*Tuesday*	*Wednesday*
ACTIVITIES			
FOCUS			
MINDFULNESS			

TRACKER	M	T	W	T	F	S	S
	○	○	○	○	○	○	○
	○	○	○	○	○	○	○
	○	○	○	○	○	○	○
	○	○	○	○	○	○	○
	○	○	○	○	○	○	○

Thursday	*Friday*	*Saturday*	*Sunday*

REFLECTIONS

JOY	CHALLENGES	MOOD	LEARNINGS

MINDFULNESS *intentions*

	Monday	Tuesday	Wednesday
ACTIVITIES			
FOCUS			
MINDFULNESS			

NOTES

TRACKER	M	T	W	T	F	S	S
	○	○	○	○	○	○	○
	○	○	○	○	○	○	○
	○	○	○	○	○	○	○
	○	○	○	○	○	○	○
	○	○	○	○	○	○	○

Thursday	*Friday*	*Saturday*	*Sunday*

REFLECTIONS

JOY	CHALLENGES	MOOD	LEARNINGS

NOTES

"Happiness is a butterfly which, when pursued is just beyond your grasp . . . but if you will sit down quietly, may alight upon you."

—NATHANIEL HAWTHORNE

MINDFULNESS
priorities

Monday	Tuesday	Wednesday

BE HAPPY IN
THE MOMENT.
THAT'S ENOUGH.

–Mother Teresa

NOTES

Thursday	*Friday*	*Saturday*	*Sunday*

BIRTHDAYS

MINDFULNESS *intentions*

NOTES

	Monday	Tuesday	Wednesday
ACTIVITIES			
FOCUS			
MINDFULNESS			

TRACKER	M	T	W	T	F	S	S
	○	○	○	○	○	○	○
	○	○	○	○	○	○	○
	○	○	○	○	○	○	○
	○	○	○	○	○	○	○
	○	○	○	○	○	○	○

Thursday	*Friday*	*Saturday*	*Sunday*

REFLECTIONS

JOY	CHALLENGES	MOOD	LEARNINGS

MINDFULNESS *intentions*

	Monday	*Tuesday*	*Wednesday*
ACTIVITIES			
FOCUS			
MINDFULNESS			

NOTES

TRACKER	M	T	W	T	F	S	S
	○	○	○	○	○	○	○
	○	○	○	○	○	○	○
	○	○	○	○	○	○	○
	○	○	○	○	○	○	○
	○	○	○	○	○	○	○

Thursday	*Friday*	*Saturday*	*Sunday*

REFLECTIONS

JOY	CHALLENGES	MOOD	LEARNINGS

MINDFULNESS *intentions*

	Monday	*Tuesday*	*Wednesday*
ACTIVITIES			
FOCUS			
MINDFULNESS			

NOTES

TRACKER

	M	T	W	T	F	S	S
	○	○	○	○	○	○	○
	○	○	○	○	○	○	○
	○	○	○	○	○	○	○
	○	○	○	○	○	○	○
	○	○	○	○	○	○	○

Thursday	*Friday*	*Saturday*	*Sunday*

REFLECTIONS

JOY	CHALLENGES	MOOD	LEARNINGS

MINDFULNESS *intentions*

	Monday	*Tuesday*	*Wednesday*
ACTIVITIES			
FOCUS			
MINDFULNESS			

NOTES

TRACKER	M	T	W	T	F	S	S
	○	○	○	○	○	○	○
	○	○	○	○	○	○	○
	○	○	○	○	○	○	○
	○	○	○	○	○	○	○
	○	○	○	○	○	○	○

Thursday	Friday	Saturday	Sunday

REFLECTIONS

JOY	CHALLENGES	MOOD	LEARNINGS

MINDFULNESS *intentions*

	Monday	Tuesday	Wednesday
ACTIVITIES			
FOCUS			
MINDFULNESS			

NOTES

TRACKER	M	T	W	T	F	S	S
	○	○	○	○	○	○	○
	○	○	○	○	○	○	○
	○	○	○	○	○	○	○
	○	○	○	○	○	○	○
	○	○	○	○	○	○	○

Thursday	Friday	Saturday	Sunday

REFLECTIONS

JOY	CHALLENGES	MOOD	LEARNINGS

NOTES

"Mindfulness means being awake. It means really knowing what you are doing."

— JON KABAT-ZINN

MINDFULNESS *priorities*

Monday	*Tuesday*	*Wednesday*

WITH THE QUIET SERENITY OF A MEDITATIVE MIND, LISTEN, ABSORB, TRANSCRIBE, AND TRANSFORM.

–Pythagoras

NOTES

Thursday	Friday	Saturday	Sunday

BIRTHDAYS

MINDFULNESS *intentions*

	Monday	*Tuesday*	*Wednesday*
ACTIVITIES			
FOCUS			
MINDFULNESS			

NOTES

TRACKER	M	T	W	T	F	S	S
	○	○	○	○	○	○	○
	○	○	○	○	○	○	○
	○	○	○	○	○	○	○
	○	○	○	○	○	○	○
	○	○	○	○	○	○	○

Thursday	*Friday*	*Saturday*	*Sunday*

REFLECTIONS

JOY	CHALLENGES	MOOD	LEARNINGS

MINDFULNESS *intentions*

NOTES

	Monday	Tuesday	Wednesday
ACTIVITIES			
FOCUS			
MINDFULNESS			

TRACKER	M	T	W	T	F	S	S
	○	○	○	○	○	○	○
	○	○	○	○	○	○	○
	○	○	○	○	○	○	○
	○	○	○	○	○	○	○
	○	○	○	○	○	○	○

Thursday	*Friday*	*Saturday*	*Sunday*

REFLECTIONS

JOY	CHALLENGES	MOOD	LEARNINGS

MINDFULNESS *intentions*

	Monday	*Tuesday*	*Wednesday*
ACTIVITIES			
FOCUS			
MINDFULNESS			

NOTES

TRACKER	M	T	W	T	F	S	S

Thursday	Friday	Saturday	Sunday

REFLECTIONS

JOY	CHALLENGES	MOOD	LEARNINGS

MINDFULNESS *intentions*

NOTES

	Monday	*Tuesday*	*Wednesday*
ACTIVITIES			
FOCUS			
MINDFULNESS			

TRACKER

	M	T	W	T	F	S	S
	○	○	○	○	○	○	○
	○	○	○	○	○	○	○
	○	○	○	○	○	○	○
	○	○	○	○	○	○	○
	○	○	○	○	○	○	○

Thursday	*Friday*	*Saturday*	*Sunday*

REFLECTIONS

JOY	CHALLENGES	MOOD	LEARNINGS

MINDFULNESS *intentions*

NOTES

	Monday	Tuesday	Wednesday
ACTIVITIES			
FOCUS			
MINDFULNESS			

TRACKER

	M	T	W	T	F	S	S
	○	○	○	○	○	○	○
	○	○	○	○	○	○	○
	○	○	○	○	○	○	○
	○	○	○	○	○	○	○
	○	○	○	○	○	○	○

Thursday	*Friday*	*Saturday*	*Sunday*

REFLECTIONS

JOY	CHALLENGES	MOOD	LEARNINGS

NOTES

"If you have your full attention in the moment, you will see only love."

—DEEPAK CHOPRA

MINDFULNESS *priorities*

Monday	*Tuesday*	*Wednesday*

WHEN I LET GO OF WHAT I AM, I BECOME WHAT I MIGHT BE.

–Lao Tzu

NOTES

Thursday	Friday	Saturday	Sunday

BIRTHDAYS

MINDFULNESS *intentions*

NOTES

	Monday	Tuesday	Wednesday
ACTIVITIES			
FOCUS			
MINDFULNESS			

TRACKER	M	T	W	T	F	S	S
	○	○	○	○	○	○	○
	○	○	○	○	○	○	○
	○	○	○	○	○	○	○
	○	○	○	○	○	○	○
	○	○	○	○	○	○	○

Thursday	*Friday*	*Saturday*	*Sunday*

REFLECTIONS

JOY	CHALLENGES	MOOD	LEARNINGS

MINDFULNESS *intentions*

NOTES

	Monday	Tuesday	Wednesday
ACTIVITIES			
FOCUS			
MINDFULNESS			

TRACKER	M	T	W	T	F	S	S
	○	○	○	○	○	○	○
	○	○	○	○	○	○	○
	○	○	○	○	○	○	○
	○	○	○	○	○	○	○
	○	○	○	○	○	○	○

Thursday	*Friday*	*Saturday*	*Sunday*

REFLECTIONS

JOY	CHALLENGES	MOOD	LEARNINGS

MINDFULNESS *intentions*

NOTES

	Monday	*Tuesday*	*Wednesday*
ACTIVITIES			
FOCUS			
MINDFULNESS			

TRACKER	M	T	W	T	F	S	S
	○	○	○	○	○	○	○
	○	○	○	○	○	○	○
	○	○	○	○	○	○	○
	○	○	○	○	○	○	○
	○	○	○	○	○	○	○

Thursday	Friday	Saturday	Sunday

REFLECTIONS

JOY	CHALLENGES	MOOD	LEARNINGS

MINDFULNESS *intentions*

NOTES

	Monday	Tuesday	Wednesday
ACTIVITIES			
FOCUS			
MINDFULNESS			

TRACKER

	M	T	W	T	F	S	S
	○	○	○	○	○	○	○
	○	○	○	○	○	○	○
	○	○	○	○	○	○	○
	○	○	○	○	○	○	○
	○	○	○	○	○	○	○

Thursday	Friday	Saturday	Sunday

REFLECTIONS

JOY	CHALLENGES	MOOD	LEARNINGS

MINDFULNESS *intentions*

	Monday	*Tuesday*	*Wednesday*
ACTIVITIES			
FOCUS			
MINDFULNESS			

NOTES

TRACKER

	M	T	W	T	F	S	S
	○	○	○	○	○	○	○
	○	○	○	○	○	○	○
	○	○	○	○	○	○	○
	○	○	○	○	○	○	○
	○	○	○	○	○	○	○

Thursday	Friday	Saturday	Sunday

REFLECTIONS

JOY	CHALLENGES	MOOD	LEARNINGS

NOTES

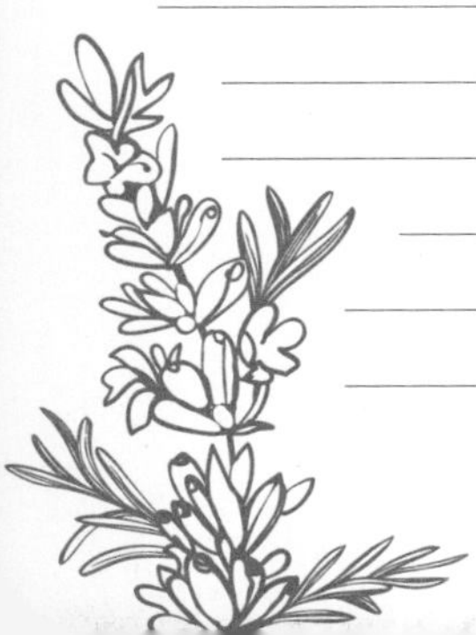

"Only when your consciousness is totally focused on the moment you are in can you receive whatever gift, lesson, or delight that moment has to offer."

—BARBARA DE ANGELIS

MINDFULNESS
priorities

THE ULTIMATE GIFT OF CONSCIOUS LIFE IS A SENSE OF THE MYSTERY THAT ENCOMPASSES IT.

–Lewis Mumford

Monday	*Tuesday*	*Wednesday*

NOTES

Thursday	*Friday*	*Saturday*	*Sunday*

BIRTHDAYS

MINDFULNESS *intentions*

NOTES

	Monday	*Tuesday*	*Wednesday*
ACTIVITIES			
FOCUS			
MINDFULNESS			

TRACKER	M	T	W	T	F	S	S
	○	○	○	○	○	○	○
	○	○	○	○	○	○	○
	○	○	○	○	○	○	○
	○	○	○	○	○	○	○
	○	○	○	○	○	○	○

Thursday	Friday	Saturday	Sunday

REFLECTIONS

JOY	CHALLENGES	MOOD	LEARNINGS

MINDFULNESS *intentions*

NOTES

	Monday	Tuesday	Wednesday
ACTIVITIES			
FOCUS			
MINDFULNESS			

TRACKER	M	T	W	T	F	S	S
	○	○	○	○	○	○	○
	○	○	○	○	○	○	○
	○	○	○	○	○	○	○
	○	○	○	○	○	○	○
	○	○	○	○	○	○	○

Thursday	*Friday*	*Saturday*	*Sunday*

REFLECTIONS

JOY	CHALLENGES	MOOD	LEARNINGS

MINDFULNESS *intentions*

NOTES

	Monday	Tuesday	Wednesday
ACTIVITIES			
FOCUS			
MINDFULNESS			

TRACKER

	M	T	W	T	F	S	S
	○	○	○	○	○	○	○
	○	○	○	○	○	○	○
	○	○	○	○	○	○	○
	○	○	○	○	○	○	○
	○	○	○	○	○	○	○

Thursday	Friday	Saturday	Sunday

REFLECTIONS

JOY	CHALLENGES	MOOD	LEARNINGS

MINDFULNESS *intentions*

NOTES

	Monday	Tuesday	Wednesday
ACTIVITIES			
FOCUS			
MINDFULNESS			

TRACKER

	M	T	W	T	F	S	S
	○	○	○	○	○	○	○
	○	○	○	○	○	○	○
	○	○	○	○	○	○	○
	○	○	○	○	○	○	○
	○	○	○	○	○	○	○

Thursday	*Friday*	*Saturday*	*Sunday*

REFLECTIONS

JOY	CHALLENGES	MOOD	LEARNINGS

MINDFULNESS *intentions*

NOTES

	Monday	*Tuesday*	*Wednesday*
ACTIVITIES			
FOCUS			
MINDFULNESS			

TRACKER	M	T	W	T	F	S	S
	○	○	○	○	○	○	○
	○	○	○	○	○	○	○
	○	○	○	○	○	○	○
	○	○	○	○	○	○	○
	○	○	○	○	○	○	○

Thursday	*Friday*	*Saturday*	*Sunday*

REFLECTIONS

JOY	CHALLENGES	MOOD	LEARNINGS

NOTES

"Life isn't about waiting for the storm to pass. It's about learning how to dance in the rain."

— VIVIAN GREENE

Monday	Tuesday	Wednesday

MINDFULNESS
priorities

THE LITTLE THINGS? THE LITTLE MOMENTS? THEY AREN'T LITTLE.

–Jon Kabat-Zinn

NOTES

Thursday	Friday	Saturday	Sunday

BIRTHDAYS

MINDFULNESS *intentions*

NOTES

	Monday	*Tuesday*	*Wednesday*
ACTIVITIES			
FOCUS			
MINDFULNESS			

TRACKER	M	T	W	T	F	S	S
	○	○	○	○	○	○	○
	○	○	○	○	○	○	○
	○	○	○	○	○	○	○
	○	○	○	○	○	○	○
	○	○	○	○	○	○	○

Thursday	*Friday*	*Saturday*	*Sunday*

REFLECTIONS

JOY	CHALLENGES	MOOD	LEARNINGS

MINDFULNESS
intentions

NOTES

	Monday	Tuesday	Wednesday
ACTIVITIES			
FOCUS			
MINDFULNESS			

TRACKER	M	T	W	T	F	S	S
	○	○	○	○	○	○	○
	○	○	○	○	○	○	○
	○	○	○	○	○	○	○
	○	○	○	○	○	○	○
	○	○	○	○	○	○	○

Thursday	*Friday*	*Saturday*	*Sunday*

REFLECTIONS

JOY	CHALLENGES	MOOD	LEARNINGS

MINDFULNESS *intentions*

NOTES

	Monday	Tuesday	Wednesday
ACTIVITIES			
FOCUS			
MINDFULNESS			

TRACKER	M	T	W	T	F	S	S
	○	○	○	○	○	○	○
	○	○	○	○	○	○	○
	○	○	○	○	○	○	○
	○	○	○	○	○	○	○
	○	○	○	○	○	○	○

Thursday	Friday	Saturday	Sunday

REFLECTIONS

JOY	CHALLENGES	MOOD	LEARNINGS

MINDFULNESS
intentions

NOTES

	Monday	*Tuesday*	*Wednesday*
ACTIVITIES			
FOCUS			
MINDFULNESS			

TRACKER

M T W T F S S

Thursday	*Friday*	*Saturday*	*Sunday*

REFLECTIONS

JOY	CHALLENGES	MOOD	LEARNINGS

MINDFULNESS *intentions*

NOTES

	Monday	Tuesday	Wednesday
ACTIVITIES			
FOCUS			
MINDFULNESS			

TRACKER	M	T	W	T	F	S	S

Thursday	*Friday*	*Saturday*	*Sunday*

REFLECTIONS

JOY	CHALLENGES	MOOD	LEARNINGS

NOTES

"Sometimes the most important thing in the whole day is the rest we take between two deep breaths."

—ETTY HILLESUM

MINDFULNESS
priorities

Monday	Tuesday	Wednesday

SMILE, BREATHE,
AND GO SLOWLY.
–Thích Nhất Hạnh

NOTES

Thursday	Friday	Saturday	Sunday

BIRTHDAYS

MINDFULNESS *intentions*

NOTES

	Monday	Tuesday	Wednesday
ACTIVITIES			
FOCUS			
MINDFULNESS			

TRACKER	M	T	W	T	F	S	S
	○	○	○	○	○	○	○
	○	○	○	○	○	○	○
	○	○	○	○	○	○	○
	○	○	○	○	○	○	○
	○	○	○	○	○	○	○

Thursday	*Friday*	*Saturday*	*Sunday*

REFLECTIONS

JOY	CHALLENGES	MOOD	LEARNINGS

MINDFULNESS *intentions*

NOTES

	Monday	Tuesday	Wednesday
ACTIVITIES			
FOCUS			
MINDFULNESS			

TRACKER	M	T	W	T	F	S	S
	○	○	○	○	○	○	○
	○	○	○	○	○	○	○
	○	○	○	○	○	○	○
	○	○	○	○	○	○	○
	○	○	○	○	○	○	○

Thursday	*Friday*	*Saturday*	*Sunday*

REFLECTIONS

JOY	CHALLENGES	MOOD	LEARNINGS

MINDFULNESS
intentions

NOTES

	Monday	Tuesday	Wednesday
ACTIVITIES			
FOCUS			
MINDFULNESS			

TRACKER

	M	T	W	T	F	S	S
	○	○	○	○	○	○	○
	○	○	○	○	○	○	○
	○	○	○	○	○	○	○
	○	○	○	○	○	○	○
	○	○	○	○	○	○	○

Thursday	*Friday*	*Saturday*	*Sunday*

REFLECTIONS

JOY	CHALLENGES	MOOD	LEARNINGS

MINDFULNESS
intentions

NOTES

	Monday	Tuesday	Wednesday
ACTIVITIES			
FOCUS			
MINDFULNESS			

TRACKER	M	T	W	T	F	S	S

Thursday	*Friday*	*Saturday*	*Sunday*

REFLECTIONS

JOY	CHALLENGES	MOOD	LEARNINGS

MINDFULNESS *intentions*

NOTES

	Monday	Tuesday	Wednesday
ACTIVITIES			
FOCUS			
MINDFULNESS			

TRACKER	M	T	W	T	F	S	S
	○	○	○	○	○	○	○
	○	○	○	○	○	○	○
	○	○	○	○	○	○	○
	○	○	○	○	○	○	○
	○	○	○	○	○	○	○

Thursday	*Friday*	*Saturday*	*Sunday*

REFLECTIONS

JOY	CHALLENGES	MOOD	LEARNINGS

NOTES

"Be happy for this moment. This moment is your life."

—OMAR KHAYYAM

Monday	Tuesday	Wednesday

MINDFULNESS
priorities

WE OWN NO PAST,
NO FUTURE, WE
ONLY POSSESS NOW.
–Mary Baker Edday

NOTES

Thursday	Friday	Saturday	Sunday

BIRTHDAYS

MINDFULNESS
intentions

	Monday	*Tuesday*	*Wednesday*
ACTIVITIES			
FOCUS			
MINDFULNESS			

NOTES

TRACKER	M	T	W	T	F	S	S
	○	○	○	○	○	○	○
	○	○	○	○	○	○	○
	○	○	○	○	○	○	○
	○	○	○	○	○	○	○
	○	○	○	○	○	○	○

Thursday	*Friday*	*Saturday*	*Sunday*

REFLECTIONS

JOY	CHALLENGES	MOOD	LEARNINGS

MINDFULNESS
intentions

NOTES

	Monday	Tuesday	Wednesday
ACTIVITIES			
FOCUS			
MINDFULNESS			

TRACKER	M	T	W	T	F	S	S
	○	○	○	○	○	○	○
	○	○	○	○	○	○	○
	○	○	○	○	○	○	○
	○	○	○	○	○	○	○
	○	○	○	○	○	○	○

Thursday	Friday	Saturday	Sunday

REFLECTIONS

JOY	CHALLENGES	MOOD	LEARNINGS

MINDFULNESS
intentions

NOTES

	Monday	Tuesday	Wednesday
ACTIVITIES			
FOCUS			
MINDFULNESS			

TRACKER

	M	T	W	T	F	S	S
	○	○	○	○	○	○	○
	○	○	○	○	○	○	○
	○	○	○	○	○	○	○
	○	○	○	○	○	○	○
	○	○	○	○	○	○	○

Thursday	*Friday*	*Saturday*	*Sunday*

REFLECTIONS

JOY	CHALLENGES	MOOD	LEARNINGS

MINDFULNESS *intentions*

NOTES

	Monday	*Tuesday*	*Wednesday*
ACTIVITIES			
FOCUS			
MINDFULNESS			

TRACKER

	M	T	W	T	F	S	S
	○	○	○	○	○	○	○
	○	○	○	○	○	○	○
	○	○	○	○	○	○	○
	○	○	○	○	○	○	○
	○	○	○	○	○	○	○

Thursday	Friday	Saturday	Sunday

REFLECTIONS

JOY	CHALLENGES	MOOD	LEARNINGS

MINDFULNESS *intentions*

	Monday	Tuesday	Wednesday
ACTIVITIES			
FOCUS			
MINDFULNESS			

NOTES

TRACKER	M	T	W	T	F	S	S

Thursday	*Friday*	*Saturday*	*Sunday*

REFLECTIONS

JOY	CHALLENGES	MOOD	LEARNINGS

NOTES

“Every time we become aware of a thought, as opposed to being lost in a thought, we experience that opening of the mind.”

— JOSEPH GOLDSTEIN

MINDFULNESS
priorities

Monday	Tuesday	Wednesday

CHANGE YOUR THOUGHTS, AND YOU CHANGE YOUR WORLD.
–Norman Vincent Peale

NOTES

Thursday	Friday	Saturday	Sunday

BIRTHDAYS

MINDFULNESS *intentions*

NOTES

	Monday	*Tuesday*	*Wednesday*
ACTIVITIES			
FOCUS			
MINDFULNESS			

TRACKER	M	T	W	T	F	S	S
	○	○	○	○	○	○	○
	○	○	○	○	○	○	○
	○	○	○	○	○	○	○
	○	○	○	○	○	○	○
	○	○	○	○	○	○	○

Thursday	*Friday*	*Saturday*	*Sunday*

REFLECTIONS

JOY	CHALLENGES	MOOD	LEARNINGS

MINDFULNESS *intentions*

NOTES

	Monday	*Tuesday*	*Wednesday*
ACTIVITIES			
FOCUS			
MINDFULNESS			

TRACKER	M	T	W	T	F	S	S
	○	○	○	○	○	○	○
	○	○	○	○	○	○	○
	○	○	○	○	○	○	○
	○	○	○	○	○	○	○
	○	○	○	○	○	○	○

Thursday	Friday	Saturday	Sunday

REFLECTIONS

JOY	CHALLENGES	MOOD	LEARNINGS

MINDFULNESS *intentions*

NOTES

	Monday	Tuesday	Wednesday
ACTIVITIES			
FOCUS			
MINDFULNESS			

TRACKER	M	T	W	T	F	S	S
	○	○	○	○	○	○	○
	○	○	○	○	○	○	○
	○	○	○	○	○	○	○
	○	○	○	○	○	○	○
	○	○	○	○	○	○	○

Thursday	*Friday*	*Saturday*	*Sunday*

REFLECTIONS

JOY	CHALLENGES	MOOD	LEARNINGS

MINDFULNESS
intentions

NOTES

	Monday	Tuesday	Wednesday
ACTIVITIES			
FOCUS			
MINDFULNESS			

TRACKER	M	T	W	T	F	S	S
	○	○	○	○	○	○	○
	○	○	○	○	○	○	○
	○	○	○	○	○	○	○
	○	○	○	○	○	○	○
	○	○	○	○	○	○	○

Thursday	Friday	Saturday	Sunday

REFLECTIONS

JOY	CHALLENGES	MOOD	LEARNINGS

MINDFULNESS *intentions*

NOTES

	Monday	Tuesday	Wednesday
ACTIVITIES			
FOCUS			
MINDFULNESS			

TRACKER

	M	T	W	T	F	S	S
	○	○	○	○	○	○	○
	○	○	○	○	○	○	○
	○	○	○	○	○	○	○
	○	○	○	○	○	○	○
	○	○	○	○	○	○	○

Thursday	Friday	Saturday	Sunday

REFLECTIONS

JOY	CHALLENGES	MOOD	LEARNINGS

NOTES

NOTES

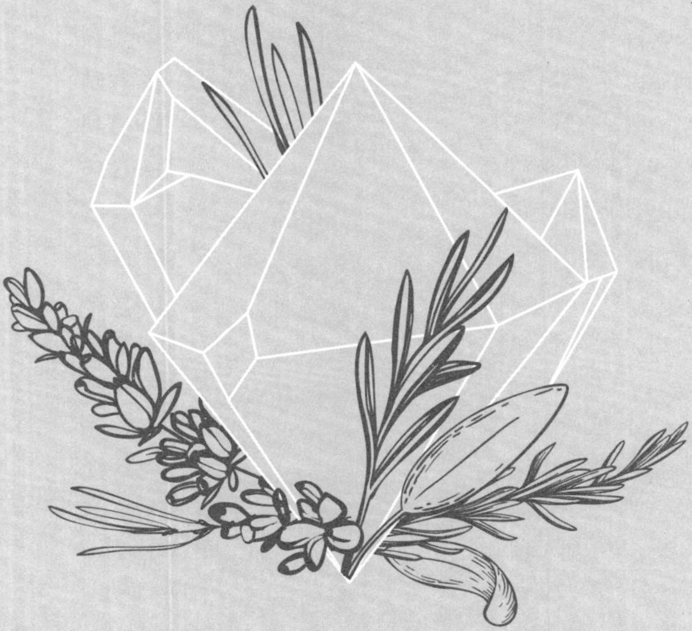

INSIGHTS

an imprint of

INSIGHT EDITIONS

www.insighteditions.com

MANUFACTURED IN CHINA

10 9 8 7 6 5 4 3 2 1